C000004270

200 MCQs in PHARMACOGNOSY

By. Dr. Betty Marshall

ISBN: 9781688234345

2019

Simple Choice

In each of the simple choice problems, only one answer is correct. Choose the correct answer.

1. The volatile oils are complex mixtures of..........
A) mono- and sesquiterpenes and phenylpropane derivatives
B) mono- and diterpene alcohols and ethers
C) sesquiterpenes and other aromatic compounds
D) monoterpene acids and lactones
E) monoterpene ethers and aldehydes

2. Which of the following are known as balsams?
A) Resins dissolved in volatile oil
B) A mixture of volatile oils with sesquiterpenes
C) Resins dissolved in water
D) Polysaccharides mixed with volatile oil
E) Juices evaporated to dryness

3. Alkaloids are naturally occurring compounds which contain ....in their molecules.
A) one or more N atoms
B) two heterocyclic rings
C) a side-chain on one of the benzene rings
D) one or more N atoms originating from amino acids
E) one or more O atoms

4. The iridoids are...
A) constituents of volatile oils
B) starting units of tannin biogenesis
C) precursors of the biosynthesis of saponins
D) precursors of the biogenesis of certain alkaloids
E) constituents of fixed oils

5. Which of the following methods is used to get alkaloids in base form from plant material?
A) Adding ammoniumhydroxide and water to the pulverized drug

B) Making an extract with mineral acid and organic solvent
C) Making an extract with base and organic solvent
D) Adding mineral acid and water to the powdered drug
E) Making an extract with organic solvent and warming it.

6. Which of the following explanations is why morphine can be separated from its accompanying alkaloids?
A) Morphine contains a piperidine ring.
B) Morphine contains two methoxy groups.
C) Morphine contains a phenolic hydroxyl group whereas the accompanying alkaloids have none.
D) Morphine does not contain phenolic hydroxyl group whereas the accompanying alkaloids contain one.
E) Morphine and its accompanying alkaloids are inseparable.

7. Which of the following is the skeleton of Cinchona alkaloids?
A) Cevan
B) Tropane
C) Isoquinoline
D) Rubanol
E) Dammarane

8. Which of the following is the reagent for alkaloids?
A) 2,4-Dinitrophenylhydrazine
B) Iron(III)chloride
C) Antimony(III)chloride
D) Potassiumtetraiodomercurate
E) Phloroglucinol in concentrated hydrochloric acid

9. Ergot is the.....................of the fungus Claviceps purpurea.
A) vegetative form
B) dried sclerotium
C) ascospore
D) conidiospore
E) filamentous hyphae

10. Which of the following is the difference between the chemical structures of cotton and starch?
A) Cotton consists of α-glucose molecules, whereas starch contains branched β-glucose residues
B) Cotton consists of unbranched β-glucose molecules, whereas starch contains unbranched α- and β-glucose residues
C) Cotton is built up from glucose residues linked by 1,4-β-D-glucose bonds, whereas starch contains branched and linear chains of 1,4-α- and 1,6-α-D-glucose residues
D) Both consist of branched and linear 1,4-α-D-glucose units
E) Both are built up from branched and linear 1,2-β-D-glucose residues

11. Which of the following is the structure of the flavonoids of Silybum marianum?
A) Dimeric flavan-3,4-diol
B) Monomeric flavon-3-ol
C) Flavonolignan
D) A simple flavanonol-glycoside
E) Isoflavanonediglycoside

12. Which of the following is the test for the identification of anthraquinones?
A) The Marquis test
B) The Froehde test
C) The Liebermann-Burchard test
D) The Borntraeger test
E) The murexide test

13. Which of the following is the way to detect procyanidins?
A) When heated with dilute NaOH, procyanidins give a green colour
B) Procyanidins give a yellow colour with concentrated nitric acid

C) When heated with cc. HCl, procyanidins give a red colour. On extraction of the mixture with nBuOH, the butanolic phase turns red

D) When heated with resorcinol, procyanidins give a bluish-violet colour

E) Procyanidins give an orange precipitate with the Kedde reagent.

14. Which of the following is the assay for determination of the volatile oil contents of herbal drugs?
A) Steam distillation
B) Extraction with light petrol
C) Distillation by Marcusson's method
D) Determination of the loss on drying
E) Determination of the alcoholic extract

15. Why is it not recommended to use Rheum raponticum instead of Rheum palmatum for medical purposes?
A) Because the emodin content of R. raponticum is too high
B) Because the rhein content of the R. raponticum is too low
C) Because the chrysophanol content of R. raponticum is too high
D) Because R. raponticum contains a stilbene derivative which has undesirable hormonal activity
E) Because the gallic acid content of R. raponticum is too low

16. Which of the following compounds transforms to chamazulen on steam distillation?
A) Lavandulol
B) Farnezol
C) Matricin
D) Gossypol
E) Parthenolid

17. Which of the following drugs contains inulin?
A) Cichorii radix
B) Symphyti radix

C) Plantaginis herba
D) Trigonellae foenugraeci semen
E) Tanaceti herba

18. Hashish is the .... of Cannabis sativa.
A) gum of the male flowers
B) resin of the female flowers
C) gum of the male and female flowers
D) pressed juice of the leaves
E) latex of the tops

19. Which of the following is opium?
A) The dried latex exudate of the unripe incised capsules
B) The dried aqueous extract of the ripe capsules
C) The dried alcoholic extract of the unripe capsules
D) A concentrated alcoholic extract of the poppy straw
E) An aqueous extract of the ripe seeds

20. Which of the following is the common skeleton of physiologically active ergoline alkaloids?
A) Isolysergic acid
B) Clavorubine
C) Lysergic acid
D) 2-Phenylbenzopyran
E) Elimoclavine

21. Poppy straw is the industrial raw material of morphine production because ...
A) poppy straw contains only morphine
B) poppy straw does not contain other accompanying alkaloids
C) poppy straw has the maximum morphine content
D) poppy straw is the cheapest available raw material
E) poppy straw contains morphine derivatives

22. Which of the following achievements is associated with Miklos Bekessy?
A) The industrial production of essential oils by steam distillation
B) The industrial production of poppy alkaloids
C) The cultivation of ergot
D) the isolation of morphine
E) The production of ergot alkaloids by fermentation

23. Which of the following drugs has the highest caffeine content?
A) Mate folium
B) Theae folium
C) Guarana
D) Coffeae semen
E) Colae semen

24. Which of the following constituents is **not** present in Matricariae aetheroleum?
A) Chamazulene
B) Matricin
C) Spatulenol
D) α-Bisabolol
E) en-in-bicyclic ethers

25. Inulin is a(n)...
A) arabin
B) pectin
C) galaktane
D) mannan
E) fructosane

26. Which of the following is an alkaloid with a purine skeleton?
A) Hygrine
B) Theobromine
C) Ephedrine
D) Strychnine

E) Solanidine

27. Which of the following drugs has a carminative effect?
A) Frangulae cortex
B) Centaurii herba
C) Silybi mariani fructus
D) Foeniculi fructus
E) Graminis rhizoma

28. Which of the following drugs contains ajoene?
A) Valerianae radix
B) Agrimoniae herba
C) Echinaceae radix
D) Ginseng radix
E) Allii sativi bulbus

29. Which of the following plant constituents can be characterized
by irreversible complexation
with proteins?
A) Alkaloids
B) Saponins
C) Tannins
D) Mucilages
E) Anthraquinone glycosides

30. Which of the following drugs contains aucubin?
A) Marrubii herba
B) Agrimoniae herba
C) Valerianae radix
D) Plantaginis lanceolatae folium
E) Cyani flos

31. Hide powder is used in the traditional method of tannin
quantitation because ...
A) hide powder gives a colour reaction with tannins

B) hide powder reacts with polyphenols
C) hide powder reduces tannins
D) hide powder oxidizes polyphenols
E) hide powder reacts with tannins

32. Which of the following types of compound is arbutin, used in urological infections?
A) A flavonoid glycoside
B) A phenolic glycoside
C) A furanocoumarin
D) An iridoid glycoside
E) A gallitannin

33. With which of the following methods can the tertiary alkaloids be extracted in salt form?
A) With organic solvents such as chloroform
B) On boiling with aqueous ammonia solution
C) With organic solvents containing alkaline solution
D) With organic solvents containing acidic solution
E) With an acidic aqueous solution

34. Which of the following drugs contains anthraquinone derivatives?
A) Betulae folium
B) Graminis rhizoma
C) Rhei radix
D) Herniariae herba
E) Rubi idaei folium

35. Which of the following reagents is suitable for identification of the Secale cornutum alkaloids?
A) The van Urk reagent
B) The Fehling I and II reagents
C) Iron(III) chloride
D) Phloroglucinol in hydrochloric acid

E) The EP reagent

36. Iridoids are...:
A) stress compounds characteristic of the Lamiaceae family
B) sesquiterpenes with a bitter taste
C) monoterpenes with a cyclopenta-(c)-pyrane structure
D) pseudoalkaloids
E) constituents of balms since they have a pleasant scent

37. The bitter value is the .... of an extract made of 1g of drug, which just has a bitter taste.
A) highest dilution
B) lowest dilution
C) lowest concentration
D) highest concentration
E) highest trituration

38. Which of the following drugs contains laxative compounds?
A) Sennae folium
B) Hyperici herba
C) Urticae radix
D) Equiseti herba
E) Agrimoniae herba

39. Which of the following is the toxic compound of linseed?
A) Arabinoxylane
B) Ricin
C) Linamarin
D) Scopoletin
E) Rhein

40. Linoleic acid is a(n)...
A) saturated ω-6 fatty acid
B) unsaturated ω-6 fatty acid
C) unsaturated ω-3 fatty acid

D) ω-9 fatty acid

E) saturated ω-3 fatty acid

41. Which of the following contains a fixed oil rich in γ-linolenic acid?

A) Zea mays

B) Sesamum indicum

C) Oenothera biennis

D) Ricinus communis

E) Glycine max

42. Which of the following compounds contains an N atom?

A) Naphthoquinone Derivatives

B) Monoterpenes

C) Coumarins

D) Lignans

E) Alkylamines

43. Atropine is a 1:1 mixture of D and L-...

A) scopoletin

B) scopolamine

C) hyoscyamine

D) belladonnin

E) scopolin

44. Which of the following "mystic" plants contains alkaloids with a tropane skeleton?

A) Betel Palm

B) Mandrake

C) Hemlock

D) Cannabis

E) Iboga

45. Which of the following indications is not applicable for Capsici fructus?

A) Topical application in rheumatic disorders

B) Stomachic
C) Promotion of wound healing
D) Relieving neuralgias
E) Increasing the rate of hair growth

46. The main compound of Ephedrae herba is the analogue of the synthetic molecule...
A) amphetamine
B) ketamine
C) phencyclidine
D) ethyl morphine
E) methadone

47. Which of the following compounds is characteristic of Rauwolfiae radix?
A) Physostigmine
B) Quinidine
C) Reserpine
D) Cytisine
E) Capsaicin

48. The comfrey root is only suitable for topical application because the drug contains ...
A) alkaloids with a tropane skeleton
B) piperidine alkaloids
C) saponins
D) pyrrolizidine alkaloids
E) coumarins

49. The toxic Conii fructus can easily be confused with...
A) fennel seed
B) linseed
C) anise seed
D) coriander seed
E) castor bean seed

50. Which of the following is the main active component of betel nut?
A) Ephedrine
B) Chlorogenic acid
C) Capsaicin
D) Hypericin
E) Arecholin

51. Which of the following types of compounds are the capsaicinoids?
A) Monoterpenes
B) Pseudoalkaloids
C) Carotenoids
D) Protoalkaloids
E) Anthocyans

52. Which of the following is the medical use of common fumitory?
A) decreasing high blood pressure
B) relieving joint pain
C) enhancing bile synthesis and excretion
D) promotion of wound healing
E) antipyretic

53. The basic structure of Boldi folium alkaloids is...
A) indole
B) piperidine
C) morphinan
D) aporphine
E) isoquinoline

54. Vinpocetine (Cavinton®) is a semi-synthetic derivative of the main active compound of which

of the following plants?
A) Rhamnus frangula
B) Pulmonaria officinalis
C) Catharanthus roseus
D) Vinca minor
E) Berberis vulgaris

55. To which of the following types of compound does taxol belong?
A) Diterpene alkaloid
B) Steroidal alkaloid
C) Sesquiterpene
D) Lignan
E) Triterpene

56. Which of the following statements relating to the traditional herbal medicinal products is false?
A) Attributing a preventive or curative effect to these products is forbidden
B) They contain one or more herbal substances, preparations or their combination as active agents.
C) The products may also contain vitamins and minerals
D) Their authorization is possible via abridged registration
E) They can be distributed in pharmacies

57. Which of the following types of medicines was developed from the alkaloid camtothecin, isolated from Camptotheca acuminata?
A) Antidiabetic
B) Anticancer
C) Hypotensive
D) Anti-inflammatory
E) Antiarrhythmic

58. Which of the following types of medicines was developed from galegine, isolated from Galega officinalis?

A) Antidiabetic
B) Anticancer
C) Hypotensive
D) Anti-inflammatory
E) Antiarrhythmic

59. Which of the following is the advantage of collecting medical herbs from their natural habitat?
A) The whole process (culturing, harvesting, etc.) can be controlled
B) The appropriate harvesting and quality can be guaranteed
C) The stock is homogeneous
D) No culturing costs are involved
E) The properties of the plants can be modified by cross-breeding

60. Which of the following groups of compounds consists of primary metabolites?
A) Alkaloids
B) Lignans
C) Flavonoids
D) Iridoids
E) Carbohydrates

61. Which of the following structural features is characteristic of saponins?
A) Their skeleton may be built up from 10, 15, 20 or 30 carbon atoms
B) They are triterpene glycosides
C) They are glycosides with aromatic rings
D) They are heterocyclic molecules containing sulphur.
E) They are mineral salts of fatty acids.

62. The essential oil of Melissa officinalis is sometimes falsified with the essential oil of...:
A) Cymbopogon winterianus

B) *Citrus aurantium*
C) *Hyssopus officinalis*
D) *Commiphora molmol*
E) *Citrus limon*

63. *Flavonoids such as … are able to decrease the permeability of the capillaries.*
A) *liquiritin and isoliquiritin*
B) *apigenin and luteolin*
C) *genistein and ononin*
D) *silybin and silychristin*
E) *hesperidin and rutin*

64. *Which of the following types of components are used in photochemotherapy (PUVA)?*
A) *Anthrone glycosides*
B) *Dimeric coumarins*
C) *Furanocoumarins*
D) *Quinoline alkaloids*
E) *Phloroglucine derivatives*

65. *Which of the following is the tetracyclic oxindole alkaloid of Uncariae tomentosae radix?*
A) *Pteropodine*
B) *Mitraphylline*
C) *Speciophylline*
D) *Rinchophylline*
E) *Theophylline*

66. *As defined by the European Pharmacopoeia, which of the following are herbal drugs?*
A) *Processed plants, plant or animal parts that are mainly used in the fresh state, or sometimes after drying*

B) Mainly unprocessed, whole or ground plants, algae, fungi or lichen, which are particularly used after drying or sometimes in the fresh state

C) Generally herbal products, prepared by different methods such as extraction, distillation, extrusion, fractionation, concentration or fermentation

D) Plant species used as therapeutic agents to influence the functions of the human body

E) Medical herbs used as therapeutic agents to influence the functions of the human body

67. Chromatography on normal-phase silica gel is based on which of the following physicochemical processes?
A) Distribution
B) Adsorption
C) Ion exchange
D) Antigen-antibody interaction
E) Thermal interaction

68. Which of the following chromatographic techniques always use forced flow?
A) Rotation planar chromatography
B) Gel-filtration chromatography
C) Thin-layer chromatography
D) Ion-exchange chromatography
E) Two-dimensional chromatography

69. Which of the following is the definition of chromatographic R_f (retention factor) value?
A) The distance that a particular compound moves from the start
B) The distance between the start and the solvent front
C) The distance that a particular compound moves divided by the distance of the solvent front from the start
D) The distance travelled by the solvent front from the start divided by the distance that a particular compound moves

E) The distance of the compound from the solvent front divided by the distance of the solvent front

70. Which of the following is the shape of maize starch grains?
A) Oval
B) Round
C) Polygonal, with a central triangular or 2 to 5 stellate cleft hilum
D) Triangular
E) Dumbbell

71. Which of the following processes can be used to prepare an extract rich in polysaccharides from linseed?
A) From grained drug with water
B) From grained drug with alcohol
C) From whole seeds with hot water
D) From whole seeds with diluted alcohol
E) From whole seeds with organic solvents

72. Which of the following is characteristic of mucilages?
A) They can be extracted from the drug with water
B) They undergo hydrolysis to monosaccharide units upon boiling
C) They can be precipitated with alcohol
D) They give a viscous solution with water
E) They can be precipitated with heavy metal ions

73. Which of the following is the main method for the preparation of fixed oils used in medicine?
A) Heating the drug with organic solvents
B) Extraction with water
C) Cold extrusion
D) Warm extrusion
E) Distillation

74. Flavonoids can be detected with reactions based on complex formation. Which of the following substituents on the flavone skeleton prevent this?
A) -OH on C5 (e.g. apigenin)
B) -OH on C3 and C5 (e.g. quercetin)
C) -O-galactoside on C5 and -OH on C3 (e.g. hyperoside)
D) -OCH$_3$ on C5 and no –OH on C3 (e.g. nobiletin)
E) -OH on C5 and -O-rutinoside on C3 (e.g. rutin)

75. Which of the following forms are alkaloids mainly present in plants?
A) Esters of mineral acids
B) Salts of mineral acids
C) Free bases
D) Esters of organic acids
E) Hydrochlorides

76. In which of the following ways can alkaloids be extracted from plants in salt form?
A) Warming with organic solvents
B) Boiling with aqueous ammonium hydroxide
C) Shaking with acidified water at room temperature or above
D) Warming with lead acetate and water
E) Shaking with acidified organic solvents

77. With which of the following tests can the alkaloids of deadly nightshade be identified?
A) The Marquis test
B) The Thalleioquin test
C) With cc. HNO$_3$
D) The Grahe test
E) The Vitali test

78. In which of the following ways is Lavandulae aetheroleum prepared?

A) Warm extrusion
B) Extraction with organic solvent
C) Warm extrusion
D) Enzyme reaction followed by extraction
E) Steam distillation

79. Which of the following is a suitable reagent for the TLC detection of carvone?
A) iodine vapour + starch solution
B) dimethylaminobenzaldehyde solution
C) vanillin-sulphuric acid
D) 2,4-Dinitrophenylhydrazine
E) 3,5-Dinitrobenzoic acid + alcoholic potassium hydroxide solution

80. Which of the following does the hemolytic index indicate:
A) The di- and sesquiterpene content of volatile oils
B) The saponin content of the drugs
C) The steroid content of the drugs
D) The aliphatic monoterpene content of volatile oils
E) The tannin content of the drugs

81. Which of the following reagents is suitable for the detection of the cardioactive glycosides of Digitalis purpureae folium?
A) 2,4-Dinitrophenylhydrazine
B) Dimethylaminobenzaldehyde solution
C) Potassium hydroxide solution
D) Iodine vapour + starch solution
E) 3,5-Dinitrobenzoic acid + sodium hydroxide solution

82. With which of the following methods can the anthraquinone derivative content of a drug be detected:
A) Upon warming of the extract with glacial acetic acid a red precipitate is formed

B) After extraction of the drug with organic solvent and mixing with diluted ammonium hydroxide solution, the separating alkaline phase shows a reddish-orange or red colour
C) The aqueous extract of the drug gives a blue precipitate with lead acetate
D) The aqueous extract of the drug forms a green complex with cc. sulphuric acid
E) The organic solvent extract of the drug gives a yellow precipitate with a mixture of dilute hydrochloric acid and chlorogen

83. Which of the following methods is specified by the European Pharmacopoeia for quantification of the anthraquinone glycoside content of drugs?
A) Gravimetry
B) High-performance liquid chromatography
C) Spectrophotometry
D) Gas chromatography
E) Titrimetry

84. Which of the following is a C-glycoside)
A) Arbutin
B) Gypsoside
C) Gentiopikrin
D) Aloin
E) Hypericin

85. Which of the following factors does **not** influence the effectiveness of chromatographic separations:
A) The polarity of the solvent
B) The humidity of the air
C) The shape of the developing chamber
D) The optical rotation of the solvent system
E) The grain size of the stationary phase

86. During steam distillation matricin breaks down. Which of the following steps is **not** involved in this process?
A) Opening of the lactone ring
B) The loss of water
C) Decarboxylation
D) Water addition
E) The loss of acetic acid

87. Which of the following drugs contains homopolysaccharide?
A) Cyamopsidis seminis pulvis
B) Acaciae gummi
C) Solani amylum
D) Agar
E) Althaeae folium et radix

88. Which of the following factors does **not** influence the effectiveness of extraction?
A) Temperature
B) The polarity of the solvent
C) The particle size of the grounded drug
D) The refractive index of the compounds to be extracted
E) The pH of the solvent

89. Which of the following volatile oils has a higher density than that of water?
A) Thymi aetheroleum
B) Caryophylli aetheroleum
C) Lavandulae aetheroleum
D) Anisi stellati aetheroleum
E) Juniperi aetheroleum

90. Which of the following is Calendulae flos?
A) A carminative
B) A cardiotonic
C) A roborant
D) An epithelogenic

E) A sedative

91. Which of the following is Silybi mariani fructus?
A) A cardiotonic
B) A roborant
C) A hepatoprotectant
D) A mild antidepressant
E) An astringent

92. Which of the following are active agents of Alchemillae?
A) Tannins (ellagic acid derivatives)
B) Alkaloids
C) Anthraquinones
D) Galaktomannans
E) Polysaccharides

93. Which of the following is the use of Alchemillae herba in medicine?
A) As laxative
B) For the treatment of eczema and skin inflammation
C) As spasmolytic
D) As hepatoprotectant
E) To increase bile production

94. Which of the following is the use of Calendulae flos in medicine?
A) To improve cognitive functions
B) As antiemetic during travel sickness
C) As spasmolytic
D) As secretolytic
E) For the treatment of skin and mucosal inflammation

95. Which of the following is the use of Zingiberis rhizoma in medicine?
A) To improve cognitive functions
B) As antiemetic during travel sickness

C) As spasmolytic
D) As secretolytic
E) For the treatment of skin and mucosal inflammation

96. Which of the following is the use of Hederae folium in medicine?
A) expectorant, secretolytic, spasmolytic
B) treatment of skin inflammation
C) cardiotonic
D) antiemec
E) epithelogenic

97. Which of the following compounds are responsible for the bitter taste of Lupuli flos?
A) Phloroglucine derivatives
B) Triterpene saponins
C) Polysaccharides
D) Pseudoalkaloids
E) Anthraquinones

98. Which of the following compounds of Hyperici herba has a photosensitizing effect?
A) Rutin
B) Hyperforin
C) Hyperoside
D) Hypericin
E) Quercitrin

99. Which of the following is the official name (specified by the European Pharmacopoeia) of the drug of bearberry (Arctostaphylos uva-ursi)?
A) Folia uvae ursi
B) Uvae ursi folium
C) Folium arctostaphylos uva-ursi
D) Arctostaphylos folium

E) *Uvae ursi folia*

100.*The volatile oil of ... is prepared by mechanical pressing (extrusion)?*
A) *Salvia officinalis*
B) *Thymus vulgaris*
C) *Quercus petraea*
D) *Citrus sinensis*
E) *Illicium verum*

The following questions have one or more correct answers. Use the notations given below:

A: *Only answer 1, 2 and 3 are correct*
B: *Only answer 1 and 3 are correct*
C: *Only answers 2 and 4 are correct*
D: *Only answer 4 is correct*
E: *All answers are correct*

101. *Which of the following drugs contain alkaloids derived from ornithine?*
1.*Nicotianae folium*
2.*Hyoscyami folium*
3.*Cocae folium*
4.*Ribis nigri folium*

102. *Which of the following properties are characteristic of tannins?*
1.*They give a precipitate with alkaloids*
2.*They give a yellow or bluish-red colour with iron(III) chloride*
3.*They transform hide into leather*
4.*They give a pale-pink precipitate with iodine*

103. *Which of the following does Hypericum perforatum contain?*

1.Phloroglucine derivatives
2.Naphthodianthrone derivatives
3.Flavonoids
4.Saponins

104. Which of the following effects do the alkaloids of
Ipecacuanhae radix have?
1.Antipyretic
2.Amoebicidal
3.Sedative
4.Expectorant

105. Which of the following plant species are steroid sources for
industry?
1.Dioscorea composita
2.Glycyrrhiza glabra
3.Smilax regelii
4.Ipomoea purga

106. Which of the following drugs contain **no** cardioactive
compounds?
1.Digitalis purpureae folium
2.Allii bulbus
3.Oleandri folium
4.Stramonii semen

107. Which of the following drugs have a high ascorbic acid
content?
1.Hippophae rhamnoides fructus
2.Manna
3.Rosae pseudofructus
4.Gallii odorati herba

108. Which of the following are the active compounds of hops?
1.Cnicine

2.Humulon
3.Loganin
4.Lupulon

109. Which of the following are treated with Ginkgo folium?
1.Concentration and memory problems
2.Restlessness, sleeplessness and anxiety
3.Dizziness and tinnitus
4.Mild cardiac insufficiency

110. Which of the following compounds are terpenoids?
1.Iridoids
2.Anthocyanidins
3.Carotenoids
4.Tannins

111. Which of the following alkaloids are bisindols characteristic of Catharanthi herba?
1.Vincristine
2.Vincamine
3.Vinblastine
4.Catharanthine

112. Which of the following herbal drugs contain sesquiterpene-γ-lactones as bitter compounds?
1.Absinthii herba
2.Centaurii herba
3.Cardui benedicti herba
4.Gentianae radix

113. Which of the following drugs containing bitter monoterpene compounds?
1.Absinthii herba
2.Cinchonae cortex
3.Marrubii herba

4.Centaurii herba

114. Which of the following alkaloid drugs play a significant worldwide role in the pharmaceutical industry?
1.Scopoliae herba
2.Catharanthi herba
3.Papaveris fructus
4.Secale cornutum

115. Which of the following drugs contain bufadienolide glycosides?
1.Scillae bulbus
2.Convallariae herba
3.Hellebori rhizoma et radix
4.Oleandri folium

116. Which of the following types of compounds are formed during the acidic decomposition of procyanidins?
1.Flavanone
2.Catechin
3.Flavonol
4.Anthocyanidine

117. Which of the following natural substances serves as starting materials in the semisynthesis of pregnenolone acetate?
1.Oleanolic acid
2.Diosgenin
3.Lanatozide C
4.Phytosterols

118. Which of the following are the basis for the distinction of Conii fructus from Anisi vulgaris fructus by microscopy?
1.Conii fructus has secretion (essential oil) ducts
2.there are no trichomes on Conii fructus

3.Anisi vulgaris fructus has no secretion (essential oil) ducts
4.Conii fructus has no secretion (essential oil) ducts

119. Which of the following drugs have an essential oil containing carvone?
1.Menthae crispae folium
2.Anisi vulgaris fructus
3.Carvi fructus
4.Menthae piperitae folium

120. Which of the following drugs have a significant carotenoid content?
1.Capsici fructus
2.Papaveris rhoeados flos
3.Calendulae flos
4.Malvae flos

121. Which of the following contain alkaloids of tropane?
1.Belladonnae folium
2.Scopoliae rhizoma et radix
3.Stramonii folium
4.Chelidonii herba

122. Which of the following alkaloids can be found in opium?
1.Papaverine
2.Noscapine
3.Thebain
4.Ephedrine

123. Which of the following compounds are characteristic of Passiflorae herba?
1.Harman
2.Pteropodine
3.Harmaline
4.Isopteropodine

124. Which of the following alkaloids belong to the ergotoxin group?
1.Ergotamine
2.Ergocristine
3.Ergostine
4.Ergocryptine

125. Which of the following plants served as starting material for the development of cytostatic medicines?
1.Catharanthus roseus
2.Helleborus niger
3.Taxus brevifolia
4.Veratrum album

126. Which of the following plants contains alkaloids of purine base?
1.Hypericum perforatum
2.Ilex paraguariensis
3.Lobelia inflata
4.Paullinia cupana

127. Which of the following drugs contain a high amount of heteropolysaccharide:
1.Plantaginis ovatae semen
2.Psyllii semen
3.Trigonellae foenugraeci semen
4.Strychni semen

128. To which of the following groups do the active agents of Ginkgo folium belong?
1.Biflavons
2.Naphtoquinones
3.Diterpenes
4.Hydroquinones

129. Which of the following are the medical uses of Echinacea drugs?
1.Reducing joint inflammation
2.Preventing the complications of respiratory tract disorders
3.Reducing digestive problems
4.They are used topically to promote wound healing

130. Which of the following drugs can be used in the treatment of benign prostate hyperplasia?
1.Silybi mariani fructus
2.Pruni africanae cortex
3.Rusci rhizoma
4.Sabalis serrulatae fructus

131. Which of the following statements relating to the Aloe species are correct?
1.Their dried juice is laxative
2.Anthraquinone derivatives are responsible for their laxative properties
3.The aloe gel rich, in polysaccharides, is stored in the parenchyma cells
4.The aloe gel can be used for the treatment of small wounds and inflammatory skin diseases

132. Which of the following pharmacognosy-related quantitative determinations are listed in the European Pharmacopoeia?
1.Determination of volatile oil content
2.Determination of 1,8-cineol content of volatile oils
3.Determination of tannin content of herbal drugs
4.Determination of the haemolytic index of herbal drugs

133. Which of the following chromatographic techniques always utilize forced flow?
1.Rotation planar chromatography

2.High-performance liquid chromatography
3.Overpressure thin layer chromatography
4.Ion-exchange column chromatography

134. Which of the following factors influence the effectiveness of extraction?
1.The temperature
2.The polarity of solvent
3.The particle size of the grounded drug
4.The method of extraction

135. During thin-layer chromatographic examination, the compound in the sample is
identical with the test compound if...
1.the sizes of the spots of the sample and test compounds are the same
2.the spots of the sample and test compounds give the same colour reaction after spraying the TLC plate with the reagent; or their colour is the same under UV light
3.the number of spots is the same in the sample and the test material
4.the compound in the sample and the test compound give the same R_f value in at least two different solvent systems

136. Which of the following are characteristic of fixed oils?
1.If used for medical purposes, they are prepared by cold extrusion
2.They are esters of glycerol
3.They are derivatives of long chain, aliphatic monocarboxylic acids, containing an odd number of C atoms
4.They are derivatives of long-chained, aliphatic monocarboxylic acids, containing an even number of C atoms.

137. Which of the following compounds are C-glycosides?
1.Arbutin

2.Vitexin
3.Gentiopicrine
4.Aloin

138. Which of the following drugs contain homopolysaccharide?
1.Lanugo gossypii
2.Gummi arabicum
3.Solani amylum
4.Agar

139. Which of the following are internal uses of Calendulae flos?
1.To treat gallbladder inflammation
2.As diuretic
3.To treat stomatitis and enteritis
4.To treat wounds

140. Which of the following are characteristic of starches?
1.They form a colloidal solution with hot water
2.They give a blue colour with dilute iodine solution
3.They are polysaccharides
4.They give a red colour with iron(III) chloride.

141. The European Pharmacopoeia prescribes HPLC methods for determination of the alkaloidcontent of which of the following herbal drugs?
1.Belladonnae folium
2.Boldi folium
3.Chelidonii herba
4.Colae semen

142. Which of the following reagents can be used for alkaloid detection?
1.The Mayer reagent
2.The Kedde reagent
3.The Dragendorff reagent

4.An alcoholic solution of 2,4-dinitrophenylhydrazine

143. The European Pharmacopeia prescribes determination of the total hydroxycinnamic acid (caffeic acid) content of which of the following herbal drugs?
1.Ballotae nigrae herba
2.Melissae folium
3.Rosmarini folium
4.Juniperi pseudo-fructus

144. Which of the following volatile oil assays are recommended in the European Pharmacopoeia?
1.Foreing esters in essencial oils
2.The residue remaining on the evaporation of essencial oils
3.The odour and taste of essential oils
4.The bitterness value

145. Which of the following volatile oils have a density higher than that of water?
1.Thymi aetheroleum
2.Caryophylli aetheroleum
3.Lavandulae aetheroleum
4.Cinnamomi cassiae aetheroleum

146. Which of the following are characteristic of tannins?
1.They give precipitates with heavy metal salts
2.They precipitate proteins irreversibly
3.They form precipitates with alkaloids
4.They do not dissolve in water or alcohol

147. Which of the following drugs contain flavonoids?
1Rhei radix
2Tiliae flos
3Aloe capensis
4Crataegi folii cum flore

148. Which of the following are medical uses of Crataegi folii cum flore?
1.As mild cardiotonic
2.As antiemetic
3.For the side-treatment of atherosclerosis and high blood pressure
4.As anti-inflammatory

149. Which of the following drugs contain hydroquinone derivatives?
1.Hederae folium
2.Myrtilli fructus
3.Salicis cortex
4.Uvae ursi folium

150. Which of the following drugs contain salicylic acid derivatives?
1.Hederae folium
2.Salicis cortex
3.Harpagophyti radix
4.Filipendulae ulmariae herba

Association

Pair each letter with the correspondent number(s).

151. A. Unsaturated fatty acids
B. Saturated fatty acids.
1.Myristic acid
2.Arachidic acid
3.Oleic acid
4. Ricinoleic acid
5. Linolenic acid
6. Palmitic acid

152. A. Chemical constituents of Allium sativum
B. Chemical constituents of Allium cepa
1. Alliin
2. Allicine
3. Diallyl-disulphide
4. Ajoen
5. Cepaen
6. Cwibelane

153. A. Compounds of Ginkgo biloba
B. after the compounds of Arnica montana.
1. Bilobetin
2. Helenalin
3. Luteolin-7-O-glucoside
4. Amentoflavone
5. Miricetin-3-O-rutoside

154. Pair the following herbal drugs with the medical uses!
A) Matricariae flos
B) Ipecacuanhae radix
C) Hyoscyami folium
D) Sennae folium
E) Capsici fructus

1.rubefacient
2.spasmolytic
3.laxative
4.parasympatholytic
5.expectorant

155. Pair the structures with the names!
A) Flavonol
B) Flavone
C) Flavanone

D) Flavane
E) Isoflavone
1. 2.
3. 4.
5.

156. Pair the herbal drugs with the medical uses.
A) Mild Sedative
B) Arthritis
C) Pharyngitis
D) Expectorant
E) Choleretic
1.Althaeae radix et folium
2.Ipecacuanhae radix
3.Uncariae radix
4.Passiflorae herba
5.Chelidonii herba et radix

157. Pair the herbal drugs with the active agents.
A) Physostigmine
B) Alliin
C) Colchicine
D) Vincristine
E) Protopine
1.Garlic
2.Common fumitory
3.Calabar bean
4.Autumn crocus
5.Periwinkle

158. Pair the compounds with the chemical structures.
A) Morphinan structure
B) Benzylisoquinoline structure
C) Tropane structure
D) Rubane structure

E) Phtalide tetrahydroisoquinoline structure
1.Scopolamine
2.Quinidine
3.Papaverine
4.Thebaine
5.Noscapine

159. Pair the drugs used in medicine with the plant species.
A) rhizoma
B) herba
C) fructus
D) cortex
E) tuber
1.couch grass
2.paprika
3.ephedra
4.cinchona
5.autumn crocus

160. Pair the drugs with the medical uses.
A) Mild laxative
B) Treatment of bruises
C) Expectorant
D) Immunostimulant
E) Alleviation of gastrointestinal spasms
1.Echinaceae pallidae radix
2.Lini semen
3.Symphyti radix
4.Chelidonii herba
5.Ipecacuanhae radix

161. Pair the drugs with the effects
A) Cytotoxic
B) Parasympatholytic
C) Muscle relaxant

D) Sympathomimetic
E) Antiplatelet
1.Belladonnae folium
2.Ephedrae herba
3.Allii bulbus
4.Curare
5.Camptotheca acuminata

162. A. Constituents of Opium
B. Constituents of Cinchonae cortex
1.Chinoic acid
2.Quinine
3.Narcotine
4.Narceine
5.Cinchonidine

163. Pair the herbal drugs with the medical uses.
A) Choleretic
B) Tonic
C) Antimalarial
D) Expectorant
E) Insomnia
1.Passiflorae herba
2.Strychni semen
3.Cinchonae cortex
4.Hederae folium
5Berberidis radix

164. A. pyrrolyzidine containing drugs
B. terpene alkaloid containing drugs
1.Veratri rhizoma
2.Aconiti tuber
3.Symphyti radix
4.Solani herba
5.Pulmonariae herba

165. Pair the herbal drugs with the active agents.
A) Ergotamine
B) Emetin
C) Cytisine
D) Tubocurarine
E) Reserpine
1.Laburni semen
2.Secale cornutum
3.Curare
4.Ipecacuanhae radix
5.Rauwolfiae radix

166. Pair the herbal drugs with the active agents.
A) Echinacoside
B) Mesaconitine
C) Viscotoxin
D) Pteropodine
E) Vitamin D
1.Monkshood tuber
2.Purple coneflower root
3.Cod liver oil
4.Common mistletoe twig
5.Cat's claw root

167. Pair the compounds with the effects.
A) Parasympathomimetic
B) Antiarrhythmic
C) Antigout
D) Uterus contracting
E) Cytotoxic
1.Quinidine
2.Colchicine
3.Pilocarpine
4.Taxol

5.Ergotamine

168. Pair the compounds originating from the same herbal source.
A) Mitraphylline
B) Cephaelin
C) Scopolamine
D) Theobromine
E) Vincristine
1.Emetin
2.Vinblastine
3.Pteropodine
4.Hyoscyamine
5.Caffeine

169. Pair the drugs with the active agents.
A) Loganin
B) Cocaine
C) Pilocarpine
D) Harmine
E) Sinigrine
1.Cocae folium
2.Strychni semen
3.Passiflorae herba
4.Jaborandi folium
5.Sinapis nigrae semen

170. Pair the plant families with the components characteristic of the species.
A) Brassicaceae
B) Solanaceae
C) Papaveraceae
D) Scrophulariaceae
E) Lamiaceae
1.Alkaloids of tropane base

2.Glucosinolates
3.Cardioactive glycosides
4.Alkaloids of morphinane base
5.Monoterpenes

171. Pair the English plant names with the Latin equivalents.
A) Guar bean
B) Cat's claw
C) Common laburnum
D) Common broom
E) Common fumitory
1.Uncaria tomentosa
2.Cyamopsis tetragonolobus
3.Laburnum anagyroides
4.Fumaria officinalis
5.Sarothamnus scoparius

172. Pair the drugs with the active agents!
A) Triticin
B) Pyrrolizidine alkaloids
C) Theobromine
D) Lobeline
E) Emetin
1.Farfarae folium et flos
2.Graminis rhizoma
3.Lobeliae herba
4.Coffeae semen
5.Ipecacuanhae radix

173. Pair the compound types with the compounds.
A) Isodianthrone
B) Heterodianthrone
C) Anthraquinone diglycoside
D) Anthrone-C-glycoside
E) Anthraquinone monoglycoside

1. Barbaloin
2. Sennoside B
3. Frangulin A
4. Glucofrangulin A
5. Rhein-rheumemodin dianthrone

174. Pair the starches with the shapes of the grains.
A) Maydis amylum
B) Solani amylum
C) Oryzae amylum
D) Tritici amylum
1. Oval or round with a central cleft or point
2. Polygonal; no cleft or striation is visible
3. Oval with eccentric striation
4. Polygonal with a central triangular or 2 to 5 stellate cleft hilum

175. Pair the drugs with the active agents.
A) Brucine
B) Ergocristine
C) Emetin
D) Quinidine
E) Scopolamine
1. Ipecacuanhae radix
2. Belladonnae radix
3. Cinchonae cortex
4. Strychni semen
5. Secale cornutum

176. Pair the glycosides with the aglycones.
A) Vitexin
B) Arbutin
C) Frangulin A
D) Rutin
E) Aloin
1. aloeemodin anthrone

2.apigenin
3.hydroquinone
4.frangulaemodin
5.quercetin

177. Pair the compounds with the assays utilized for their identification.
A) Morphine
B) Scopolamine
C) Ergotoxine
D) Quinine
E) Caffeine
1.Vitali test
2.Murexide test
3.Thalleioquin test
4.van Urk test
5.Marquis test

178. Pair the herbal drugs with the assays utilized for their identification.
A) Murexide test
B) Vitali test
C) Borntraeger test
D) Rubremetin test
E) Baljet test
1.Frangulae cortex
2.Digitalis purpureae folium
3.Ipecacuanhae radix
4.Theae folium
5.Belladonnae folium

179. Pair the English and Latin names of the plant parts.
A) Rhizome
B) Flower
C) Root

D) Seed
E) Fruit
1.Semen
2.Flos
3.Rhizoma
4.Fructus
5.Radix

180. Pair the English and Latin names of the plant parts.
A) Fruit
B) Bark
C) Pericarp
D) Shoot
E) Pomaceous Fruit
1Herba
2Fructus
3Pseudo-Fructus
4Cortex
5Pericarpium

181. Pair the compounds with the assays utilized for their identification.
A) Marquis test
B) van Urk test
C) Vitali test
D) Murexide test
E) Thalleioquin test
1.Quinine
2.Scopolamine
3.Ergotamine
4.Morphine
5.Caffeine

182. Pair the herbal drugs with the assays utilized for their identification.

A) Murexide test
B) Vitali test
C) van Urk test
D) Thalleioquin test
E) Marquis test
1Papaveris fructus
2Coffeae semen
3Cinchonae cortex
4Secale cornutum
5Hyoscyami folium

183. Pair the herbal drugs with the medical uses.
A) Sinapis nigrae semen
B) Sabalis serrulatae fructus
C) Harpagophyti radix
D) Carvi aetheroleum
E) Centellae asiaticae herba
1.Treatment of benign prostate hyperplasia
2.Rubefacient
3.Carminative
4.Treatment of second- and third-degree burns
5.Anti-inflammatory

184. Pair the herbal drugs with the medical uses.
A) Melaleucae aetheroleum
B) Pini silvestris aetheroleum
C) Centellae asiaticae herba
D) Curcumae xanthorrhizae rhizoma
E) Lupuli flos
1.Sedative, hypnotic
2.Antifungal
3.Chronic venous insuffitiency
4.Expectorant
5.Amarum

185. Pair the herbal drugs with the medical uses.
A) Sinapis albae semen
B) Plantaginis lanceolatae folium
C) Cynarae folium
D) Absinthii herba
E) Calendulae flos
1.Amarum
2.Epithelogenic
3.Rubefacient
4.Treatment of upper respiratory tract diseases
5.Hepatoprotectant

186. Pair the herbal drugs with the effect.
A) Agni casti fructus
B) Orthosiphonis folium
C) Silybi mariani fructus
D) Caryophylli floris aetheroleum
E) Melissae folium
1.Hepatoprotectant
2.To decrease the prolactin hormone level
3.Anxiolytic
4.Disinfectant and local anaesthetic
5.Diuretic

187. Pair the herbal drugs with the active agents.
A) Sinapis nigrae semen
B) Harpagophyti radix
C) Centellae asiaticae herba
D) Silybi mariani fructus
E) Allii sativi bulbus
1.S-containing peptides
2.Flavonolignans
3.Iridoid glycosides
4.Triterpenes
5.Glucosinolates

188. Pair the herbal drugs with the active agents.
A) Caryophylli floris aetheroleum
B) Gentianae radix
C) Lupuli flos
D) Cimicifugae radix
E) Ononidis radix
1.Isoflavonoids
2.Triterpenes of cycloarthenol type
3.Phloroglucine derivatives
4.Secoiridoid glycosides
5.Eugenol

189. Pair the herbal drugs with the medical uses.
A) Pruni africanae cortex
B) Ononidis radix
C) Liquiritiae radix et rhizoma
D) Hippocastani semen et cortex
E) Allii bulbus
1.Treatment of chronic venous insufficiency
2.Expectorant
3.Against the development of atherosclerosis
4.Diuretic
5.Treatment of benign prostate hyperplasia (phases I and II)

190. Pair the herbal drugs with the active agents.
A) Hederae folium
B) Liquiritiae radix et rhizoma
C) Crataegi folii cum flore
D) Hyperici herba
E) Uvae ursi folium
1.Naphtodianthrone derivatives
2.a-Hederin
3.Glycyrrhizinic acid
4.Procyanidins

5.Arbutin

191. Pair the herbal drugs with the effects.
A) Allii sativi bulbus
B) Lavandulae flos
C) Carvi fructus
D) Eleutherococci radix
E) Myrtilli fructus recens
1.Antiplatelet agent
2.Tonic
3.Sedative
4.To ameliorate the microcirculation dysfunctions in the eye
5.Carminative

192. Pair the herbal drugs with the active agents.
A) Alchemillae herba
B) Podophylli rhizoma
C) Allii sativi bulbus
D) Lavandulae flos
E) Uvae ursi folium
1.Linalool
2.Lignans
3.Arbutin
4.Ajoen
5.Tannins

193. A. Drugs containing salicylic acid derivatives
B. Drugs containing hydroquinone derivatives
1.Salicis cortex
2.Uvae ursi folium
3.Vitis idaeae folium
4.Violae herba cum flore
5.Filipendulae ulmariae herba

194. A. Drugs containing phenyl propane derivatives

B. Drugs containing coumarins
1.Cinnamomi cortex
2.Levistici radix
3.Meliloti herba
4.Caryophylli floris aetheroleum
5.Rutae herba

195. A. Drugs containing iridoid glycosides
B. Drugs containing sesquiterpene derivatives
1.Tanaceti parthenii herba
2.Harpagophyti radix
3.Plantaginis lanceolatae folium
4.Absinthii herba
5.Agni casti fructus
6.Cynarae folium

196. A. Drugs containing iridoids
B. Drugs containing sesquiterpene derivatives
1.Gentianae radix
2.Chamomillae romanae flos
3.Verbenae herba
4.Matricariae flos
5.Millefolii herba
6.Plantaginis lanceolatae folium

197. A. Products of primary metabolism
B. Products of secondary metabolism
1.Polysaccharides
2.Alkaloids
3.Fixed oils
4.Terpenoids
5.Peptides and proteins
6.Phenolic compounds

198. A. Properties of gums

B. Properties of starches
1.Heteropolysaccharides
2.Produced in higher plants as a protective agent after injury
3.Homopolysaccharides
4.Built up from amylose and amylopectin
5.Constituents of dusting powders

199. Pair the Latin and the English names of the plant species.
A) Symphytum officinalis
B) Helianthus tuberosus
C) Vitex agnus castus
D) Serenoa repens
E) Hypericum perforatum
1.Jerusalem artichoke
2.Comfrey
3.Saw palmetto
4.Monk's pepper
5.St. John's wort

200. Pair the drugs with the active agents
A) Berberine
B) Protopanaxadiol
C) Glycyrrhizin
D) Cinnamaldehyde
E) Inulin
1.Cichorii radix
2.Chelidonii herba
3.Liquiritiae radix
4.Ginseng radix
5.Cinnamomi cortex

Keys

Simple Choice

1. A	32. B	63. E
2. A		64. C
3. D	33. E	
4. D	34. C	65. D
5. C	35. A	66. B
6. C	36. C	67. B
7. D	37. A	68. A
8. D	38. A	69. C
9. B	39. C	70. C
10. C	40. B	71. C
11. C	41. C	72. B
12. D	42. E	73. C
13. C	43. C	74. D
14. A	44. B	75. B
15. D	45. C	76. C
16. C	46. A	77. E
17. A	47. C	78. E
18. B	48. D	79. D
19. A	49. C	80. B
20. C	50. E	81. E
21. D	51. D	82. B
22. C	52. C	83. C
23. C	53. D	84. D
24. B	54. D	85. D
25. E	55. A	86. D
26. B	56. A	87. C
27. D	57. B	88. D
28. E	58. A	89. B
29. C	59. D	90. D
30. D	60. E	91. C
31. E	61. B	92. A
	62. A	93. B

94. E	113. D	132. A
95. B	114. C	133. A
96. A	115. B	134. E
97. A	116. C	135. C
98. D	117. C	136. A
99. B	118. C	137. C
100. D	119. B	138. B
101. A	120. B	139. B
102. B	121. A	140. A
103. A	122. A	141. C
104. C	123. B	142. B
105. B	124. C	143. A
106. C	125. B	144. A
107. B	126. C	145. C
108. C	127. A	146. A
109. B	128. B	147. C
110. B	129. C	148. B
111. B	130. C	149. C
112. B	131. E	150. C

Association

151. 1–B, 2–B, 3–A, 4–A,5–A
152. 1–A, 2–A, 3–B, 4–A,5–B
153. 1–A, 2–B, 3–B, 4–A,5–A
154. 1–E, 2–A, 3–D, 4–C,5–B
155. 1–D, 2–A, 3–E, 4–B,5–C
156. 1–C, 2–D, 3–B, 4–A,5–E
157. 1–B, 2–E, 3–A, 4–C,5–D
158. 1–C, 2–D, 3–B, 4–A,5–E
159. 1–A, 2–C, 3–B, 4–D,5–E
160. 1–D, 2–A, 3–B, 4–E,5–C
161. 1–B, 2–D, 3–E, 4–C,5–A
162. 1–B, 2–B, 3–A, 4–A,5–B
163. 1–E, 2–B, 3–C, 4–D,5–A
164. 1–B, 2–B, 3–A, 4–B,5–A
165. 1–C, 2–A, 3–D, 4–B,5–E

166. 1–B, 2–A, 3–E, 4–C,5–D
167. 1–B, 2–C, 3–A, 4–E,5–D
168. 1–B, 2–E, 3–A, 4–C,5–D
169. 1–B, 2–A, 3–D, 4–C,5–E
170. 1–B, 2–A, 3–D, 4–C,5–E
171. 1–B, 2–A, 3–C, 4–E,5–D
172. 1–B, 2–A, 3–D, 4–C,5–E
173. 1–D, 2–A, 3–E, 4–C,5–B
174. 1–D, 2–C, 3–B, 4–A,
175. 1–C, 2–E, 3–D, 4–A,5–B
176. 1–E, 2–A, 3–B, 4–C,5–D
177. 1–B, 2–E, 3–D, 4–C,5–A
178. 1–C, 2–E, 3–D, 4–A,5–B
179. 1–D, 2–B, 3–A, 4–E,5–C
180. 1–D, 2–A, 3–E, 4–B,5–C
181. 1–E, 2–C, 3–B, 4–A,5–D
182. 1–E, 2–A, 3–D, 4–C,5–B
183. 1–B, 2–A, 3–D, 4–E,5–C
184. 1–E, 2–A, 3–C, 4–B,5–D
185. 1–D, 2–E, 3–A, 4–B,5–C
186. 1–C, 2–A, 3–E, 4–D,5–B
187. 1–E, 2–D, 3–B, 4–C,5–A
188. 1–E, 2–D, 3–C, 4–B,5–A
189. 1–D, 2–C, 3–E, 4–B,5–A

190. 1–D, 2–A, 3–B, 4–C,5–E
191. 1–A, 2–D, 3–B, 4–E,5–C
192. 1–D, 2–B, 3–E, 4–C,5–A
193. 1–A, 2–B, 3–B, 4–A,5–A,
194. 1–A, 2–B, 3–B, 4–A,5–B, 6–A
195. 1–B, 2–A, 3–A, 4–B,5–A, 6–B
196. 1–A, 2–B, 3–A, 4–B,5–B, 6–A
197. 1–A, 2–B, 3–A, 4–B,5–A, 6–B
198. 1–A, 2–A, 3–B, 4–B,5–B,
199. 1–B, 2–A, 3–D, 4–C,5–E

200. 1–E, 2–A, 3–C, 4–B,5–D

Printed in Great Britain
by Amazon

24320458R00037